Upgrade Your Medical Practice's Bottom Line!

10 Ways to Decrease Costs, Increase Cash Flow, Add a New Revenue Stream and
THRIVE!

John Elliott Churchville, Ph.D., J.D.
Nancy-Ellen Churchville

New Revenue Stream Solutions
An imprint of Churchville Triad Consulting Group

Copyright © 2017 by John Elliott Churchville

All rights reserved. No part of this book shall be reproduced or transmitted in any form or by any means, electronic, mechanical, magnetic, photographic including photocopying, recording or by any information storage and retrieval system, without prior written permission of the publisher. No patent liability is assumed with respect to the use of the information contained herein. Although every precaution has been taken in the preparation of this book, the publisher and author assume no responsibility for errors or omissions. Neither is any liability assumed for damages resulting from the use of the information contained herein. Although the author is an attorney, he is not providing legal advice of any kind in this book. Readers are urged to seek their own legal counsel to answer any legal questions that may be raised in their specific situations by the general non-legal advice contained herein.

Cover design: Nancy-Ellen Churchville

ISBN-13: 978-1977624079

ISBN-10: 1977624073

BISAC: Medical/Practice Management and Reimbursement

This book is dedicated to all the women and men who have dedicated their lives to the healing profession, but especially to those who have focused their medical practices on serving the primary healthcare needs of families—children, adolescents, adults and seniors.

TABLE OF CONTENTS

Introduction

Adopt Outsourced Medical Claims Management   1

Store Medical Records in the Cloud   6

Offer Patients a Payment Plan Option   10

Handle Past-Due Patient Collections Gently   13

Set Up an Automated Patient Follow Up System   14

Prepare for RAC Audits in Advance   15

Switch to Web-Based Document Management   17

Keep a Physician Toolbox™ on Hand   19

Install a Turn-key Allergy Lab in Your Office   20

Comply with HIPAA and MACRA Rules   23

Receive a Free Medical Practice Analysis   30

About Churchville Triad Consulting Group   31

Introduction

If you know about my work on behalf of people considered last, least and lost in American society, or have read any of my books, or heard any of my talks, then you are wondering how a guy with my activist background and radical social views about liberation of the oppressed and economic justice for the poor would ever team up with and offer services and assistance to—of all people—medical doctors!

My reasons are really quite simple. I fought for the civil rights of African Americans as a voter registration worker in Southwest Georgia and a teacher of adult literacy in the Delta of Mississippi during the early 1960s because we were underdogs. I became an educator and was founder and headmaster of a private independent school for inner city at-risk youth in Philadelphia, PA, from the mid-1960s to the late 1970s because they were underdogs. I became a financial services professional providing personal, business planning and Registered Investment Advisory services to middle class workers who were facing an uncertain future in the turbulent 1980s because they were underdogs. In 1990 I became a lawyer and practiced the craft for over 25 years because my business clients were underdogs.

I earned a Ph.D. in religious studies and taught controversial courses in *African American Theology* and *African American Church History* to mainline seminary students in order to challenge their thinking about the *status quo* religion that they were being trained to serve up to underdogs. I published 14 books, established community development corporations and engaged in HIV/AIDS community outreach, testing and connection to continuum-of-care projects that were all addressed to underdogs.

1f you haven't figured out yet where I'm going with this, I'll tell you plainly: *I have teamed up with medical doctors because in the United States in the 21st century, medical doctors are true underdogs and need help to get out of that status as quickly as humanly possible.*

Everyone else thinks that you have it made, but you and I know better. You work harder over longer hours than almost anyone else. You have carried, and may still be carrying the debt of the world on your shoulders as you struggle to meet family obligations, stay abreast of your professional responsibility to maintain excellence in patient-centered care and meet the onerous demands of constantly changing governmental regulations. What is amazing is that you are able to accomplish all of this within a demanding business model that you neither fully control nor were you ever trained or equipped to handle in medical school or during your residency. If what you live and struggle through cannot be defined as underdog status, then I don't know what can!

I ask that you suspend your disbelief for a few minutes and embrace the inconvenient truth that you are an underdog who needs all the help that this mini-book can offer you. There are ten (10) ways offered here to upgrade your practice: 1) Adopt outsourced medical claim filing; 2) Store medical records in the Cloud; 3) Offer patients a payment plan option; 4) Handle past-due patient collections gently; 5) Set up an automated patient follow up system; 6) Prepare for RAC audits in advance; 7) Switch to web-based document management; 8) Keep a Physician Toolbox™ on hand; 9) Install a turn-key allergy lab in your office; and 10) Comply with HIPAA and MACRA rules.

If you are able to implement these practice-modernizing suggestions, even if only to test their efficacy, then I can make a bold and daring promise to you: you will be able to abandon your underdog status and begin to thrive not just financially, but emotionally, psychologically and spiritually as well.

Whatever *prosperous* may mean to anyone else, to you it must mean getting out from under mountains of debt and responsibility that do not help you serve the healthcare needs of your patients, and being able to thrive now and retire later to a stress-free lifestyle that you have more than earned by your diligent labor and personal sacrifice. The theologian in me cannot resist the temptation to be transparent and express my own personal concern for and empathy with you in biblical language: "My heartfelt prayer for you, my very dear friend, is that you may be as healthy and prosperous in every way as you are in soul."
(3 John 2 PHILLIPS)

John Elliott Churchville
Managing Partner
Churchville Triad Consulting Group

1: Adopt Outsourced Medical Claims Management

The first and foremost step you must take in order to decrease costs and increase revenue in your medical practice is to outsource your medical claim filing. But you cannot afford to outsource that aspect of your practice to anyone. You must do your due diligence and find a third-party vendor who is reputable, reliable and resourced sufficiently in order to effectively and timely handle your business and guarantee the shortest time span between submission of a claim to a payor and your receipt of that related payment from the payor. In addition, the third-party vendor's charges to your practice for services rendered should be totally eclipsed by the payments your practice receives.

The only way those charges can be eclipsed is if the vendor can guarantee a payment rate on claims submitted to payors to be in the range of not less than 98%. In short, this means that the vendor must be able to guarantee that at least 98% of the claims submitted will be paid—i.e., the service rendered will vastly exceed the customary average 30% denied/pended claim rate so common in the overwhelming majority of medical claims cases.

It is imperative that your practice connect with such a vendor and not settle for anyone or anything less. As you seriously consider this suggestion, you become immediately aware that making a change in this area will be quite disruptive of your current office practices. You are absolutely right! All change is disruptive. That is why most people fight change tooth and nail! The best way to assess whether a particular change is worth the bother is to test whether it leaves you with more benefits than deficits. So, let's go there!

The first step in assessing whether to make a change in how your practice is currently handling its claims is to have a Practice Analysis done. This is where you look closely at key indicators of where your practice is financially. You'll want to look carefully at the time span between when you provide services to patients and when the claims associated with your services are actually submitted to the payor. *The American Health Insurance Plans* (AHIP) has found that 29% of claims were received from health care providers more than thirty (30) days after the service was provided.

You'll want to know the average of your practice's Days Sales Outstanding (DSO). *The AHIP Center for Policy and Research* has estimated that the typical medical office has a DSO of 52 days, and more than 20% of their A/R balance is 120+ days out. Another aspect of the Practice Analysis is to discover the average percentage of practice claims submitted that are rejected. *The American Academy of Professional Coders* reported that the average number of rejected claims for a medical practice is around 34%. *The Academy Coding Edge* reported that 25-40% of rejected claims are never resubmitted for payment.

Because medical diagnostic and procedure codes are constantly changing to adapt to both medical innovations and regulatory changes, the Practice Analysis must examine the extent to which coding practices are keeping up with these changes. In a recent study undertaken by *Physician Practice Options*, it was found that 80% of all doctors undercode, 15% overcode, and only about 5% code accurately.

The purpose of a Practice Analysis is to assess the extent of financial leakage problem areas in the practice so that they can be fixed sooner, rather than later. The *New England Journal of Medicine* recently reported that 24 cents of every dollar coming into a medical practice is wasted on administrative and billing expenses. That's nearly 25% of a practice's income that goes to needless expenses—you can't afford to have that situation in your medical practice!

You are already doing your practice claims filing in-house or by a third-party billing company. If you're using in-house personnel, you may be concerned about having to let these faithful workers go. If you're using a third-party vendor, you're concerned about whether the transition will be worth the effort it takes to make it. (As my grandmother would put it, "You need to find out whether getting the juice is worth the effort you have to use to squeeze the fruit!")

Although the results of the Practice Analysis should dictate the course of action your practice will take, let's address concerns related to having to let staff go first. This is a particularly sensitive area because the livelihoods of people you know and trust are at stake. Your first priority as a physician is to excel in providing healthcare services to your patients. After this comes your responsibility to treat your staff fairly and have them treat you fairly as well. Billing staff members who do not "work their EOBs" are treating your practice unfairly because they do not see the necessity of resolving every issue that arises out of pending and denied claims. On the other hand, if billing staff are engaged in other office work (although this is rarely the case) that keeps them from "working their EOBs," then by outsourcing those duties staff can better concentrate on the other duties they must perform. Instead of losing good employees, you are repositioning them to be more productive in the areas your practice needs them most.

As you think of your best billing staff members, consider repurposing them in your practice. Who might become an excellent MA or LPN? Whose people skills might place them on the front desk or otherwise reposition them to serve as patient service reps? There is also the option of referring them to a billing company or a colleague who needs a good biller. As for those who are not producing the results the practice needs, parting company and relieving the practice of paying wages without receiving comparable results is very much in order.

We can now address the issue of replacing the current third-party billing vendor who is unable to achieve a 98% return on claims submitted to payors. If you can be assured of a 98% return on claims, then releasing the current third-party billing vendor is a no-brainer.

When considering your new third-party billing vendor, there are several key points to keep in mind that go beyond the 98% return rate. Does the vendor use Cloud-based technology so that patients' records are not stored on their computers, opening up the possibility for violating HIPAA compliance rules related to patient confidentiality? Does the vendor give the physician direct and continuing access to claim status data in real time? Are timely reports available to the physician without having to go through the vendor to get them? These are all important questions that must be answered to your satisfaction.

Unfortunately, there are too many practicing physicians who have virtually no idea about what is going on in their practice financially until it's time to bring the accountant in for tax returns at the end of the year. The 21st century thriving medical practice must have instant access to its financial data in real time at any moment. This is necessary so that adjustments can be made in a timely fashion to maximize the practice's income, decrease costs/expenses and thereby increase its net revenues in every area of operations.

2: Store Medical Records in the Cloud

More and more, paper files, folders and the furniture and fixtures that house them are becoming obsolete. As physician practices begin to plan and implement their electronic health record (EHR) conversion strategy, they realize that the choices are overwhelming and the cost to make the transition seems discouraging. However, the transition doesn't have to be as complicated, costly and painful as it appears. Many small to medium size medical practices are finding web-based EHR systems to be the perfect solution for their clinical needs. But answering the question of what kind and which EHR system to use can be vexing.

There are two kinds or categories of EHR systems on the market: cloud-based and client-server. On the one hand, a cloud-based system stores a practice's data on external servers and can be accessed via the web, requiring only a computer with an Internet connection. Client-server systems, on the other hand, store data in-house, requiring a server, hardware and software installed in the physician's office. While in-house servers have traditionally been the norm, medical practices are increasingly switching to the cloud for at least five (5) extremely good reasons.

First, implementation is much simpler with cloud-based EHR systems because EHR software runs on the web instead of the computer, meaning there are no hardware or software installations within the practice. Practices can prevent interruption of cash flow and get a faster return on investment with an implementation process much quicker than traditional client-server systems. In addition, with the right EHR system, the practice does not have to update software or hardware because of coding or regulation changes because all HIPAA-compliant updating is done by the vendor providing the service.

Second, practices realize tremendous savings from cloud-based EHR systems. One of the largest hurdles for small medical practices is the initial cost of EHR installation. Client-server systems can cost $40,000 or more just to get set up, and then the licensing fees, maintenance costs, updates and patches cost more on top of that. Since cloud-based EHR requires no hardware installation or software licenses, implementation is a fraction of the cost. Practices pay a monthly fee, like a utility bill, as part of an arrangement called Software as a Service (SaaS).

Third, IT resource requirements are significantly reduced when practices choose to move medical records to the cloud. Instead of requiring a team of IT experts to install, configure, test, run, secure and update hardware and software, all of that is done internally in the cloud by the SaaS provider. Updates are also done automatically in web-based systems, so practices are running on the most up-to-date version available.

Fourth, web-based software provides superior accessibility and collaboration over client-server systems because users are able to securely log in to the system from anywhere they have Internet connection. The ability to access the system outside of the office allows physicians, staff and patients to collaborate more effectively in a secure environment and provide better continuity of care.

Fifth, scalability is simplified with cloud-based systems. Small practices are able to expand without the standard IT growing pains. A web-based EHR system makes it easy to add new users, doctors or locations. The flexibility of web-based software allows small practices to think big and grow without breaking the bank.

A major concern of most physicians who are skeptical of cloud-based EHR systems is their feeling that security of practice and patient data might be at risk. While uncertainty is understandable, web-based EHR systems can actually deliver greater security than client-server systems and paper records.

Web-based EHR systems achieve HIPAA compliance through data centers with bank-level security and high-level encryption methods that render data unreadable—even if a security breach occurs. Client-server systems are often left unencrypted and are only as secure as the room where they are stored.

The bottom line is that cloud-based data is safer than paper and client-server records in the event of a natural disaster or fire because the data is backed up securely in multiple locations. Back-ups for client-server records are most vulnerable to breach in transport to storage facilities, unlike cloud systems.

Most people are already allowing a great deal of their sensitive data to be stored in the cloud. Email systems like Gmail and Yahoo! are stored in the cloud. Online banking, shopping and personal information on social sites like Facebook are all cloud-based systems as well.

Ultimately, cloud-based EHR systems provide users of all sizes and industries great advantages in cost savings, data accessibility and security. So, if your medical practice has not already done so, store your practice's medical records in the cloud!

3: Offer Patients a Payment Plan Option

As a healthcare provider, you know all too well how consumerism has affected your practice's bottom line. As high-deductible plans become more common and patients are responsible for a larger portion of their healthcare costs, physician practices are finding it more difficult to collect the full portion of the patient responsibility.

But the rise in healthcare costs also has a direct effect on patient health, as patients who are struggling to pay medical bills are opting to prolong treatment. A recent study by The Kaiser Family Foundation found that among respondents who had trouble paying medical bills, 31% said having trouble paying medical bills caused problems with getting other needed care. Delaying treatment, however, can exacerbate healthcare costs because by the time patients ultimately do seek care, they are sicker and treatment is more expensive.

As health insurance premiums continue to grow (at an average annual rate of 7.1 percent [AHIP 2010]), employers are switching to lower cost, high-deductible health plans. This trend is resulting in an overall decrease in payor payments and a consequent increase in patient payments. This will likely continue throughout the next decade as Congress tries to figure out how to amend, delete or otherwise replace the Affordable Care Act, one way or the other. As a result, medical practices are more dependent on patients for revenue.

To collect more from patients, some practices have started to use patient-centered strategies, such as payment plans. However, to improve results and increase efficiency, medical practices need to ensure that they are using the most efficient methods to get the desired result—collection of outstanding patient bills without disruption of the doctor/patient relationship.

There are two approaches that practices use for this purpose: the manual approach and the automated approach. In terms of the manual approach to patient collections, data from the 2011 "Trends in Healthcare Payments" report shows that the use of payment plans for healthcare payments has doubled since 2009. In the same report, 63% of surveyed patients said that they would utilize payment plans for their healthcare bills if given the option.

Many medical practices support payment plans manually by enlisting billing services to manage a calendar that shows when each payment is owed and by calling patients to collect every month. This method is a step in the right direction, but it adds to the billing service's work effort, does not ensure payment for the medical provider, and has security flaws. Whether the payment plan is set up while the patient is in the office or after a statement is sent, billing services and medical practices should securely collect and store payment information so they can automatically collect payments when they are due.

Even when a patient authorizes automated monthly payments, he or she may still forget about the payment until it shows up on their next statement, which may create confusion and costly charge-backs. In order to improve communication and offer payment transparency, all email notifications to patients prior to each payment transaction should be automated.

In order to help your patients get the care they need—and ensure you get paid what you are owed, you should seek to partner with a company to offer patient payment plans. These programs allow patients to apply for zero interest loans for out-of-pocket healthcare costs. The programs are designed to be no-risk for patients, offering easy signup and flexible payment terms.

For participating providers, patient payment plans allow them the opportunity to receive guaranteed payment—at a reduced percentage—shortly after the patient visit. This improves cash flow and reduces the administrative costs associated with trying to collect from patients. The provider is also not held responsible if the patient doesn't repay the loan.

Given all the above, there is one patient payment plan that we highly recommend to medical practices because of its automated nature and low cost to implement. It is a web-based service that gives patients the option to pay balances they owe the doctor via a Web Based Patient Portal in full or in smaller installments. Payments can be made by Debit or Credit Card and there are no volume requirements. This ideal system includes the Web Based Patient Portal and is a much lower cost option than traditional collection services. It integrates with most Practice Management Software. Doctors rave about the increased revenue from this service and how it has freed their staff from the drudgery of chasing patient balances. Some practices have seen a 100% increase in patient payments using the service and love the convenience and privacy it affords patients. Features include: 1) Web-based; 2) works with any browser on any platform; 3) integrates with other systems; 4) customizable to integrate with the practice's website; 5) convenient payment options that include Debit or Credit Card.

4: Handle Past-Due Patient Collections Gently

One of the most delicate issues facing the medical practice is collecting past-due amounts from patients. In this situation, the medical practice should engage a service that automatically collects past-due accounts via requests for payment—not threats of litigation.

It is also important that the service communicate to the medical provider the "why" of patient failure to pay which may be due to the patient's physical health. In every step of the collection process, good will and patience must be extended so that the doctor/patient relationship remains strong and does not degenerate into an adversarial one.

5: Set Up an Automated Patient Follow Up System

Doctors are regularly losing patients due to lack of an efficient follow-up system. That's where a completely automated web-based system that sends out check-up reminders, birthday cards, holiday cards, etc. to patients comes in.

The system sends out personalized full-color postcards and greeting cards that are printed and sent through the US Postal System (not e-cards). Patients are entered once into the online contact manager, and the system does the rest. Your practice can schedule Campaigns to go out automatically monthly. The system that I recommend has 18,000 pre-designed greeting card and postcards for your practice to choose from and personalize. The system allows photos to be added and can even scan in the doctor's signature and place it on each card to give it that personalized look. Signatures can be printed in blue ink to look even more "real" and you have a choice of fonts, colors, etc. to personalize each card as you wish.

6: Prepare for RAC Audits in Advance

One of the services that we recommend to doctors is to prepare—in advance—for audits by Recovery Audit Contractors (RAC) with whom the U.S. Government has contracted to go into healthcare facilities and audit their claims. Their purpose is to determine if Medicare overpaid for procedures, and to see if they agree with medical determination of diagnoses and treatments. These audits have recovered more than $300 million dollars in three years.

This service engages Certified Medical Coders to review practice records and includes preparing an audit report and a personal review of the report with the physician. This is a valuable service to medical practices because it allows Certified Medical Coders to do a baseline audit, or review of a random sample of patient files.

These Professional Coders have extensive experience in coding as well as government audits. Their provision of a detailed, comprehensive base-line audit review in advance of the actual RAC Audit is intended to assist the provider in identifying and correcting errors in the current billing and coding, and to make recommendations for areas of improvement. By catching errors well in advance, a practice can save thousands of dollars in Medicare overpayments. The cost of doing an independent review, independent of Medicare, is minimal when you consider that not knowing what the audit contractors are going to find could cost doctors thousands in penalties and loss of revenue.

In addition, up to 15% of all providers may find that they are being underpaid by Medicare due to improper coding. Medicare is not only looking to recover money, but to pay back underpayments as well. This service pinpoints these underpayments by Medicare and allows the practice to resubmit claims for correction. This has increased revenue up to 30% for some practices.

7: Switch to Web-Based Document Management

There are a number of web-based document management systems in the marketplace. But we have found one that we have unequivocally recommended to the medical practices that we serve.

iDocsNow™ is a secure web-based platform specially designed to transition any organization from managing hard copy paper records to a state-of-the-art electronic document system. Built on web-based Internet technology, iDocsNow™ requires no additional software, hardware, space or support personnel. This platform enables your medical practice an extremely usable, high performance, secure and accessible product with a quick and easy implementation and deployment schedule.

iDocsNow™ is an electronic document management solution allowing organizations to securely scan, capture, retrieve and view documents from any Internet connection in a simple, cost-effective manner. iDocsNow™ works in concert with virtually any IT system, allowing quick, seamless integration. It has unlimited scalability making it ideal to provide benefits to smaller sized organizations with a handful of critical users and equally suitable to larger enterprise-wide deployments with hundreds of employees who need worldwide access.

Project access and specific functionality limitations result in maximum control with extensive security level options for user groups. The features of this system include: 1) HIPAA compliant audit logs and reports of all user and document activity; 2) management of work queues; 3) ability to scan, view, print, route and store medical charts; 4) simple, user-friendly web-based application interface; 5) immediate deployment; 6) secure encrypted platform; 7) unlimited, full-time access to file documents; 8) access to IT support, help-desk and administration services; 9) ability to grant temporary, limited, secure access to external users; and 10) simple, user-friendly web-based application interface.

8: Keep a Physician Toolbox™ on Hand

The PhysicianToolbox™ is a proprietary suite of third-party services designed to meet the operational needs of the medical practices that we serve. The suite contains services such as transcription, credentialing, automated lab results hotline and continuing education. Members of the American Business Systems Network of independent Certified Medical Revenue Managers make this service available to the medical practices they serve so that they can serve as their one point of contact to address any need that may arise in their practices.

9: Install a Turn-key Allergy Lab in Your Office

One sure way that primary care physicians, pediatricians, and family practices can bring in a new revenue stream is by having a turn-key allergy testing and customized immunotherapy treatment lab installed right in their office. As the generalist who has already created a patient-centered medical home for your patients, your practice has the opportunity to provide a new service that brings in additional income without having to incur any capital costs at all—now or ever.

We heartily recommend BioTek Labs as the company that can offer you a turn-key testing and treatment operation that will meet this new revenue stream expectation.

BioTek Labs is a national ancillary services provider dedicated to building long-lasting relationships with medical group practices to improve existing patients' quality of life by desensitizing environmental airborne allergies. They provide managed, turn-key allergy testing and treatment labs and customized immunotherapy treatment protocols within already established medical group practices.

BioTek Labs has been delivering allergy testing and treatment services since 2004. Its Medical Director is Stuart Rusnak, MD, a Pediatric Allergist.

Having opened well over five hundred (500) labs nationwide and still counting, BioTek Labs are located primarily in the Southeastern United State, Western states and in New York State. Now they have expanded to the Eastern states.

The major immediate benefit your practice will receive from BioTek Labs is that they will provide all equipment and supplies and a fully-trained MA or LPN. In exchange, your office must supply at least a 10' x 10' or larger room that locks, has no carpet on the floor or wall covering (in order to meet OSHA standards), phone/internet access and sharps biohazard disposal service. While all charges will go through a third-party billing company having expertise in allergy diagnostic and immunotherapy procedure codes, all payments will come directly to your practice.

BioTek Labs will invoice the practice twice monthly for the agreed-upon fair market value of services provided. (The arms-length written Service Agreement contract between BioTek Labs and your practice will not run afoul of the Stark law or the safe harbor provisions of the Anti-Kickback statute.)

The addition of the allergy lab in your office will benefit your patients immensely because it enhances the continuity of care for your patients, follows the patient-centered treatment model and is financially beneficial.

Continuity of care for your patients includes their comfort, access and convenience. Patients already have an established relationship and trust built with their primary care providers. Access becomes important when it can take months before your patients can get on an allergist's schedule. (There are fewer than 4,000 allergists and more than 50 million allergy sufferers in the U.S.) Convenience for your patients is evident when they can have insurance verifications and testing performed the same day as a regular office visit and receiving results within 20 minutes. In addition, they will make fewer office visits than they would if they were using the typical allergist's model of treatment.

The patient-centered treatment model used by BioTek Labs significantly reduces office visits—instead of going to an allergist's office every month, they come to your office every other month. A second aspect of patient-centered treatment is that the initial dose and ramp-up doses of the customized allergy treatment protocol are performed in your office under observation every two months. While in the office, patients are taught how to self-administer maintenance dosing every other day in the comfort of their own homes. (For children and adolescents, parents or guardians are trained on how to administer maintenance dosing for their children.)

The in-house treatment of patients' allergies is financially beneficial to patients because: 1) nearly all insurances cover the program; 2) 70% of carriers waive deductibles; 3) there are no specialty co-pays; 4) immunotherapy is the ONLY treatment that changes the underlying disease process by effectively treating the disease; and 5) patients no longer have to buy over-the-counter medications.

The addition of a BioTek Labs allergy testing and treatment office within your office benefits your practice as well in five specific ways. First, it provides your patients with another service under your roof. Second, you get to oversee another aspect of your patients' healthcare. Third, your practice gains patients' confidence by being a more effective advocate of their overall health. Fourth, your practice can attract new and retain existing patients by offering this additional service. Fifth, your practice provides an option to underserved populations with limited access to specialty care.

If at least 4% of the patients that come to your practice present with allergy symptoms, then you should seriously consider having a BioTek Lab installed in your office.

10: Comply with HIPAA and MACRA Rules

HIPAA (Health Insurance Portability and Accountability Act of 1996) specifies rules and regulations for the protection and use of Personal (or Protected) Health Information (PHI) which is essentially a patient's medical record. What is HITECH (Health Information Technology for Economic and Clinical Health Act)? In 2010, the Act was passed in order to update HIPAA rules and provided federal funds for deploying electronic medical records (EMR), also referred to as electronic health records (EHR). HITECH upgraded HIPAA because medical records were now in digital form, and as a result, they needed new rules for protection and availability.

What does HIPAA cover? HIPAA covers the Privacy, Security and Enforcement rules of PHI. The Privacy and Security rules contain information on how one must treat PHI (whether it's electronic or not). The enforcement rules specify the penalties for failure to treat PHI properly.

There are three things that HIPAA requires: 1) Integrity of information—The medical record must be accurate; 2) Confidentiality—The medical record should only be seen by those with a need to know and all uses of that data should be knowable by the individual; and 3) Availability—The medical record must be available, in essence, with no reasonably avoidable downtime.

Why do these Acts exist? HIPAA was intended to ease the sharing of Personal Health Information (PHI) between entities that have a need to know while maintaining an acceptable and reasonable level of privacy to the individual whose information is at stake. HITECH was intended to fund and define sharing rules for Electronic Medical Records (EMR) to further their use in hopes of curtailing growing health care costs.

Who's in Charge? The Acts are administered by the Department of Health and Human Services (HHS) or the Office of Civil Rights (OCR). It is the OCR which has the right to enforce, audit, fine and charge companies and individuals for violations of the Act. They interpret the law in the Act and write the rules and regulations.

What are the rules and regulations? The rules and regulations are documented in the Code of Federal Regulations (CFR). Parts 160 and 164 of the CFR are the two that pertain to HIPAA. When someone says they adhere to HIPAA rules, it means they adhere to the paragraphs in those parts. For example, one of the paragraphs reads: "Paragraph 164.308(a)(1)(i) Standard: Security Management

Practices—Implement policies and procedures to prevent, detect, contain, and correct security violations." This means that the standard for measurement of compliance is not input—i.e., what a medical practice documents that it has done (e.g., designated a Compliance Officer, made sure that staff was trained, etc.). Rather, compliance is demonstrated by outcomes—i.e., the medical practice provides OCR with measurable results from the policy actions it has taken. Failure to show measurable outcomes is grounds for OCR penalties being imposed on the practice.

Health care is going through tremendous reform. Legislative requirements are continuing to evolve. As a result, it is imperative for health care organizations to have a partner they can trust. Contact us to find out how your medical practice can simply and cost effectively Achieve, Illustrate and Maintain HIPAA, HITECH and Omnibus Compliance.

We turn now to MACRA-related (Medicare Access and CHIP Reauthorization Act) rules—particularly those under MIPS (Merit-Based Incentive Payment System) that became law in 2015 but required medical practices to be on-board during 2017. We begin by examining the Quality Payment Program (QPP).

The Quality Payment Program implements provisions of the Medicare Access and CHIP Reauthorization Act of 2015 (MACRA) and improves Medicare payments to focus on care quality for patients.

The Quality Payment Program combines and replaces three separate Medicare related programs with a single system where Medicare clinicians have the opportunity to be paid more for doing what they do best—making their patients safer and healthier. The vast majority of measures in the program are clinician-initiated, ensuring that Medicare is rewarding what matters most to clinicians and their patients.

You are a part of the MIPS track of the Quality Payment Program if you bill Medicare Part B more than $ 30,000 as an individual clinician and provide care for more than 100 Medicare Part B patients during the determination period, and are a physician, physician assistant, clinical nurse specialist or certified registered nurse anesthetist.

You do not participate in MIPS if you are: 1) in your first year of enrollment as a Medicare provider; 2) below the low-volume threshold (care for 100 or fewer Medicare beneficiaries or have $30,000 or less in Medicare Part B allowed charges in a year); 3) above the threshold for significantly participating in an Advanced APM (Advanced Alternative Payment Models).

You were given the opportunity to pick your pace for the Quality Payment Program. You could choose to start anytime between January 1 and October 2, 2017. Whenever you chose to start, you were required to send in your performance data by March 31, 2018.

If you did not participate by October 2, 2017, then in order to avoid being penalized beginning January 1, 2019, you must report *something*—even if it relates to one patient and one performance area—for 2017 by the March 31, 2018 due date.

If you decide to participate in an Advanced APM, you may earn an incentive payment through Medicare Part B. If you decide to participate in MIPS, you will earn a performance-based payment adjustment—up, down, or not at all—based on the data that you submit.

In either track, the first payment adjustments based on performance in 2017 go into effect on January 1, 2019.

In 2017, you could assess your readiness and decide how and when you'd participate in MIPS. Your options included: 1) submitting the minimum amount of 2017 data required to Medicare and avoiding a negative payment adjustment; 2) submitting a minimum of 90 days of 2017 data to Medicare to earn a neutral to positive payment adjustment; and 3) submitting up to a full year of data to earn a positive payment adjustment.

If you didn't submit any 2017 data, then you will receive a negative 4% payment adjustment beginning January 1, 2019!

In order to decide how you want to participate, choose whether you want to submit data as an individual or as part of a group. Individual clinicians are identified by a unique combination of his or her individual National Provider ID (NPI) and Tax ID Number (TIN). Clinicians who assigned their Medicare billing rights to a group organizational TIN can submit their data either: 1) as part of a group TIN, pooling all clinicians' data; or 2) as an individual.

Choose your submission mechanism and verify its capabilities. You can submit data via: 1) Qualified Clinical Data Registry (QCDR); 2) Electronic health record (EHR); 3) Qualifying registry; 4) Claims; or 5) CMS web interface.

Be sure to verify your EHR vendor or registry's capabilities before your chosen reporting period. Contact your EHR vendor or registry directly to verify their reporting deadlines and confirm that they will be able to report your data to CMS.

Next, choose your measures and activities and pick your pace. On QPP.CMS.GOV, you can sort by specialty and data submission mechanism to choose measures that work best for you and your practice.

When selecting measures, consider the clinical conditions you treat, where you practice, your practice improvement goals, and quality information you may submit to other payers.

Be sure to review your current billing codes and Quality and Resource Use Report to help identify measures and activities that best suit your practice. Also, verify the information you need to report successfully. Each measure may require different elements and different reporting periods. Please make note of the elements and reporting period that apply to the measures you choose.

Care for patients and record data. Collect data as you care for your patients. Submit your data by March 2018 to avoid a negative payment adjustment.

Finally, if the HIPAA and MACRA compliance rules required of you and your practice seem overwhelming, then don't despair. We can and will help you with all of your compliance needs.

Receive a Free Practice Analysis

The most efficient and effective first step for your practice to take to discover whether or not it should implement any of the changes we have suggested is to engage us to perform a free, no obligation Practice Analysis. The purpose and function of the Practice Analysis is to use your data to both pinpoint areas where costs can be saved and provide solutions for increasing your practice's cash flow.

As revenue cycle management consultants, Churchville Triad Consulting Group is equipped to provide this free service to you and then—if you choose—to implement every single suggestion offered in this mini-book.

About Churchville Triad Consulting Group

Churchville Triad Consulting Group is a company that specializes in training, coaching and providing support to entrepreneurs in the healthcare industry. From this knowledge base and vantage point, we are positioned to help medical practices become more profitable by decreasing their expenses, increasing their revenue and providing them a new source of revenue.

Our **Mission** to physicians is to add value to their medical practices by helping them to decrease operational costs, increase cash flow and develop new revenue streams so that they can concentrate on growing their practices by focusing their full attention on delivering optimum healthcare outcomes for their patients.

Our **Vision** for physicians is to become the catalyst that empowers medical practices to grow beyond economic viability and sustainability to thrive as they expand their practices and the scope of patient-centered healthcare services to their current and future patients.

Our **Core Values** are those embodied in the acronym **C.R.A.D.L.E.**

Collaboration: We will achieve our business goals by working cooperatively with our clients and championing their right to expect and receive nothing less than excellence in the goods and services we provide them;

Respect: We will treat each client, employee and business associate with deference;

Acceptance: We will always be open to serving all persons with whom we do business;

Diversity: We embrace racial, ethnic, nationality and cultural differences and view these as critical factors for our company's growth and development;

Legacy: When our work for clients is completed, we will leave behind integrity, prosperity and good will;

Energy: Principled investments in our personal relationships with clients will propel us to sustainable, long-term profitability.

The Team

John Elliott Churchville, Ph.D., J.D.
Summary of Experience:

- 25 years as a practicing attorney in business law, corporation and non-profit start-ups and commercial law
- Infrastructure development for business and social entrepreneurs
- Leadership and business coaching, and internal organizational development
- Motivational speaker and Managing Partner of Churchville Triad Consulting Group

Nancy Ellen Churchville
Summary of experience:

- 25 years of healthcare industry experience
- Medical Billing/Coding Systems Analyst-5 years (Seimens)
- Medical Billing/Coding Instructor-5 years (1199C Training and Upgrading Fund)
- Medical Billing/Coding Supervisor-10 years (Hospital of the University of Pennsylvania)

- Medical Billing/Coding Specialist-5 years (Hahneman University Hospital)

Dirk Davis
Summary of Experience:

- An entrepreneur, business coach, motivational speaker and President of Mayday Physician Management Services
- 12 years experience in healthcare related services

Vicki Rackner, MD
Summary of experience:

- Retired surgeon and clinical faculty at the University of Washington School of Medicine
- Entrepreneur who translates the world of medicine into understandable strategies and tactics that are critically important to engage physicians
- Nationally noted expert, author and speaker who draws from her experience in owning her own medical practice and dealing with billing professionals

Terrence C. Patterson, M.Ed., MHA
Summary of experience:

- Involved in Healthcare Administration for over twenty years
- Guided the development of hundreds of employees in the insurance and healthcare industries, working with Blue Cross Blue Shield of Massachusetts, United Health Plans of New England and Delta Dental of Massachusetts

Jeanette Weiler, CPC
Summary of Experience:

- Certified Professional Coder, member of the American Academy of Professional Coders who has over 25 years of practice management, coding, auditing and billing experience

Marc Haskelson
Summary of Experience:

- President and CEO of Compliancy Group, a company founded in 2005 by former auditors and HIPAA compliance experts that has helped thousands of clients **Achieve, Illustrate and Maintain™** total HIPAA, HITECH, Omnibus and Meaningful Use compliance.

www.ingramcontent.com/pod-product-compliance
Lightning Source LLC
Chambersburg PA
CBHW050029230526
45470CB00003B/1189